Keys to Weight Loss Success

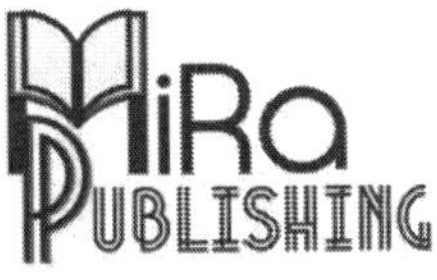

Portsmouth, VA

Keys to Weight Loss Success

Make THIS time THE Time
You Reach Your Weight Loss Goals

Rachael Watson

MiRa Publishing

Unless otherwise noted, all Scripture quotations are from the King James Version of the Bible.

Printed in the United States of America

Table of Contents

Acknowledgements

First and foremost, I want to thank God for loving me enough to intervene in my life and challenge me to get my weight under control. For pushing me to develop the discipline I need to finally make THIS time THE time I reached my goal. I love you Lord!

I want to thank my husband Michael for his support, love, encouragement, push, motivation, coaching, cooking and cheers. Thank you for hiding the snacks from me so that I don't get tempted! I love you and appreciate your help, support and sacrifice to allow me to walk in the call of God for my life.

I thank my daughter, Mikayla, for being my "trainer". For all the time you sacrifice to allow Mommy to work out and work on the vision, I love and appreciate you.

I thank my daddy, Johnny Clemons, for setting the example of weight loss for me. I watched you transform your body and your health, and you set the standard for me. Thank you for being the trailblazer. I love you and am proud of you!

I thank my mom, Bessie Clemons, for being so excited and proud of me that you pushed me into being accountable. Without you, this time would have been like all the other times. Thank you for your love, support, and encouragement to tell me that I could be and do anything I put my mind to. You were right! I Love you!

To my boys, Jason, Michael, Trinity, and Tre, I LOVE you guys so much! You are my inspiration, my joy and my heart. I pray nothing but God's greatest and best blessings on your lives!

I thank my Pastor, Apostle Despina Marie. You looked within me and saw all that God had planned and you pushed me beyond myself so that I could give birth to God's vision. Without you, Fitness Finesse w/Rae would not exist! Thank you for ALL that you have done to support me, Michael, Mikayla and MiRa! I am proud of the success that you have accomplished as the Fitness Finesse with Rae Accountability Group Poster Child! You have made THIS time THE time you reach your goals and indeed, your latter years shall be greater than your former! Love you!

To the Fitness Finesse w/Rae Accountability Group: I appreciate you guys so much!!! You have kept me accountable and on track. Thank you for trusting me and allowing me to help you reach your goals. I KNOW that each of you CAN do it! You WILL make THIS time THE time your reach your goals! There is NOTHING you cannot do! You can do ANYTHING you put your mind to! All you have to do is get your head in the game! You've got this and I LOVE YOU!!! You guys ROCK!!

To all those that have succeeded on this journey and left an example for me to see, I appreciate you for not giving up. You may not have known I was watching, but I was, and your journey encouraged, inspired and motivated me to know that it was possible and to keep going! Thanks so much!!!

Introduction

The battle to lose weight is prevalent on many minds. Many have tried and failed, or tried and succeeded only to gain the weight back eventually. I am no different. I too am in both of those categories. However, in February 2013, I started a journey that would change the course of my life. I have lost and kept off over 40 pounds and have reached my first goal weight, getting back to my wedding day dress size. This has been an amazing journey for me because I still marvel that I have reached this place and have been able to keep it off. My journey has and continues to inspire many others to do the same, and for that I am grateful.

My goal with writing this book is to share some elements that I have found to be my keys to success. Without these things, I would have yet another time of trying, but not achieving or maintaining my goal. We all know that we have to eat right and exercise, those are givens. However, there are many other factors that play a part in achieving success. These are the mental, social, and emotional factors that are crucial to success. So you will not find a diet plan or exercise routine in this book, but you will find these "keys" listed and explained, as well as my personal story related to each.

It is my passion to help people find victory in this area. As I continue my journey to my ultimate goal, I want to help share what I have learned along the way. Be encouraged! I know the challenge; I understand the struggle first hand. I know it is not easy, but it is SO worth it! Trust me, if I can do it...ANYBODY CAN DO IT!!!

My Story

I have struggled with my weight for as long as I can remember. I was always chubby or "thick". I started and stopped diets and exercise regimens, losing then regaining more weight than I lost many times in my life. By December 2012, I tipped the scales at 247 pounds. This was the heaviest I had ever been in my life and given my track record, I was subconsciously afraid to start another diet for fear of gaining even more back if I stopped again. I was afraid this would be an endless cycle until I reached 300 pounds, and I was really at a loss.

My husband and I had our annual physicals scheduled for January, and I decided that when I went, I would ask our doctor for weight loss help/advice, nutrition classes, etc. I had started taking some herbal pills that were supposed to help curb appetite, but I really felt I needed medical intervention at this point. During my appointment, I asked my doctor for some help in losing weight. He went on to tell me that he had been recommending a pill to his patients for the last year and half, but that the only person that had successfully lost weight on it had actually ended up gaining back more than he lost after one year. He was really at a loss for what to suggest, as that had been his "go to" answer. He stated that basically, over a lifetime, women gain and lose so much weight that they screw their metabolism up and in his exact words, as a 40-year-old woman, "you're pretty much stuck with it unless you workout like a dog".

Well, needless to say, I left out of there a little deflated and more discouraged. However, there was something in his words that made me want to prove him wrong. There was a resolve in my mind as I processed his words that refused to let me take them to heart. Now, let me say that I have never had any negative words come from my doctor before, and I really love him. He's a great doctor. I just figure he was having a bad day …or maybe I just needed to be challenged by his words…either way; I was determined to prove him wrong.

I started thinking about diets that I had heard about, and I knew I could do it because I had done it so many times before. I knew how to lose weight; I just needed to do what it took to lose it. That was the hard part, getting my body and appetite to line up with my determination. I would always do well at first, but when the cravings began to hit, I would always mess up…how would this time be any different?

It took a few days for me to process everything; what he said, where I was, where I wanted to be, and I began thinking about a new diet program. Well, in the meantime, my husband's physical was scheduled for a couple of days after mine. As I was still continuing to research, he went to his appointment. He was diagnosed as pre-diabetic. See he too had reached his heaviest weight as well, weighing in at 269 pounds. He left the doctor's office that Friday determined that he would lose his weight as well. Well, this diagnosis was the blessing that I needed because now, we were both on a mission! See, in times past, I would always be the one trying to work out and lose weight while my husband was not on the same journey. This was hard for me because he is a snacker. He always has snacks on his nightstand: cookies, candy, snack cakes, chips, etc. So, while I would be trying to lose weight, in a moment of weakness, I would think about the taste of that snack in my mind, and I would reach over and say, "Let me get some of those". His form of support and assistance on my journey would be to say something like, "Bae, you know you're trying to lose weight", and I would give him the look of death as if to say, "Don't tell me what I'm trying to do…I KNOW what I'm trying to do…just hand it over Bub!!!"

So now, we were on the same journey, same mission, same focus…NOW maybe I could be successful in this weight-loss journey. On the way home from this appointment, I was inspired and excited and determined to find a weight-loss regimen that we could employ. Over the weekend, I thought about the NutriSystem Diet, and remembered that they used the glycemic index to prepare their foods, and that this is the eating plan that many diabetics have to use. I started doing research and the more I looked, the more complicated it became; but I was determined that I would take the time to figure it out because I HAD to lose this weight. Well, the following Monday morning, my life would change forever. I was downstairs preparing to get my workday started, and my husband yelled to me, "Bae, come see this!!!" I said, "What is it?" He said, "There is a doctor on TV that has created this diet that you can lose two dress sizes in six weeks and you can do it eating hamburgers!" Well, that's all he had to say! I ran upstairs to see what the doctor had to say. Well, it was Dr. Ian Smith, and he was talking about the Shred Diet that he had created and just published. He was saying that you could lose two dress sizes and four inches in six weeks. He was saying that you could eat hamburgers occasionally, pancakes and pizza, as they were a part of the program as well. I was SOLD, and I rushed to purchase my copy of it on the Internet that day. We reviewed the program, and we started the next day.

By the end of those 6 weeks, I lost 18 pounds and was in a 14/16-dress size (I started at an 18/20). It was a great way to jump-start my weight-loss journey. Well, at the time of this writing, it is over a year-and-half later, and I have lost over 40 of the 80 pounds I am working to lose and have gone from a size 18 to a size 12/14. My goal is a size 10 and weight of 165 pounds. I've never been that size before, so I am excited to reach that goal.

I've learned some things along this journey that I have found to be the *Keys to Success* in a weight loss journey, and they have nothing to do with the type of food you eat or the exercises you do. So, I have written this book to encourage those of you out there that may be like me, that may feel like you will never lose the weight, that you'll never be successful and that your lot in life is just to be satisfied being a "Big Girl or Guy". Know that being big is not your lot in life, unless you choose it to be. You don't have to be BIG anymore. If I can successfully lose and maintain that weight-loss…ANYONE can do it…TRUST ME!!!! However, it starts with you. Are you ready to use your keys to unlock the New You? Then let's get started!

Chapter One
Key #1: Mindset

Dictionary.com defines mindset as the ideas and attitudes with which a person approaches a situation, especially when these are seen as being difficult to alter. Being overweight and the thought of the effort that it takes to lose that weight may seem like a difficult situation to alter. However, you have to have a "defining moment" that will trigger your goal of losing weight and committing to making the changes that are necessary to begin that journey.

My defining moment was not just one moment, but three moments that spanned a month's time. In December 2012, I had been on a fast with my husband wherein we were only drinking water and eating no food. My first defining moment was roughly around the fourth day as I climbed upstairs to get something from our room. As I was walked up those steps, I became more fatigued and breathed heavier with each step. As I reached the top, I stood there for a moment to catch my breath. I pondered why it was so hard for me to do something that had not taken nearly as much energy to do before that moment. As I stood there contemplating, I realized my energy was depleted due to the lack of food. I made a statement to God and said, "Wow Lord, I didn't realize how food energizes our bodies". As soon as those words left my mouth, I heard a response from Him. He said, "Yes, food was given to you as fuel for your body, not to fluff it. You must fuel your body and not fluff it". This experience, plus my doctor's visit and my husband's subsequent doctor's visit all tied into the desire to begin my quest to lose weight.

What is your defining moment? What is that spark that you need to jolt you into the determination that you need to do what you need to do, beyond what you feel like doing, in order to start this journey? I've started an accountability group for the individuals that are embarking upon their journey, and one of the young ladies told me that her motivation was for her husband and children. It wasn't enough motivation for her to want it for herself, but she had a defining moment that opened up the possibility of what would happen to her family if she were ill, or God-forbid, no longer here. This was the jolt that she needed. You have to have that motivation, that thing that will help you realize that THIS is the time to do it and that ***THIS*** time will be ***THE*** time you reach your goal. If you have not had that yet, but you know that you need it, I would suggest that you pray and ask God to give it to you.

Your Defining Moment

What does that defining moment do for you? It helps you get in the mindset that you need to get in. Once your mind is made up, there is nothing you can't do. Your mind has to be "all in" in order for the rest of you to commit to this journey. Changing habits, lifestyle, and behaviors is NOT easy! It is the challenge of a lifetime, but it is possible. It takes determination, consistency, effort, hard work, commitment, and focus. You have to keep your eyes on the prize and in the face of temptation, be of the mindset that you are not going to let anything deter you from your desired objective. That can only come from a mind that is determined to achieve your goal.

Personally, I have found that I can do anything I set my mind to. When I first hear a directive from the Holy Spirit that I need to consecrate or fast, my appetite begins to whine and complain immediately. It is not until my mind fully processes what is required and then commits to it that I can do it, but when I commit mentally, I have found that I don't have any problems with the fast at all. I can go for days without eating when my mind is on board, and I don't have any problems with headaches, nausea, hunger pangs, cravings, etc. When I commit, I can resist everything that comes my way. If I yield mentally by giving attention to the craving, I start having issues; even if I don't eat, my mind begins to focus on when I can eat again, and I am struggling the rest of the way. It's that mental focus; commitment, dedication, and determination that are needed to stand in this weight-loss journey. If you can get that level of commitment, then you have already won over half the battle. The victory starts in your mind first.

Know this, your body will be kicking and screaming! It will want to do what it has always done, but you are going to have to tell it what you are going to do and not the other way around. See, we have trained our bodies to be undisciplined, and now we have to train them to be disciplined. There is a scripture in the bible that God would use to motivate me. It is Proverbs 25:28, "*He that hath no rule over his own spirit is like a city that is broken down and without walls.*" The walls of a city are its defense and protection. If it has no walls, it is open and vulnerable to attack. Well, it is the same way in our bodies. If we have no control over ourselves, then we open ourselves up to all kinds of consequences. Speaking specifically about our eating, we open ourselves up to obesity, diseases, detrimental conditions, etc. We must exercise discipline and control over our appetites to protect ourselves from the detrimental consequences that can result from a lack of it.

Albert Einstein is quoted as having given the definition of insanity as: "Doing the same thing over and over again, yet expecting a different result." If we continue to do what we've always done, we will continue to get the same results that we've always obtained. Why would we think a different result would come from that? So, if we want to see change, we must change the way we think and change our mindsets. We retrain our bodies and our appetites to exhibit and respond to self-control and self-discipline.

When we have a craving that is not a part of our eating regimen, we must resist! It will seem like it's the hardest thing you've ever had to do in your life, but you MUST SAY NO!

Create a Vision

You must create a vision of who you want to be, where you want to be, and what you want to look like. If you're trying to get back to a weight you used to weigh, then find a picture of yourself back then and keep it before you. If you're trying to reach a weight you've never reached before, then cut out a picture of someone that is your desired size, and put your head on the body! That may sound funny, but having a visual helps to keep you focused on what you're working towards. Look at that vision daily, or envision yourself at that goal daily.

I remember when I was 25-years-old; I had just gotten my best job at that point in my working career. I had my own office overlooking the river and I was making $30,000 a year. One day, not long after I started, I sat down at my desk and as I was sitting in the seat, I had an open vision. I saw myself in a plush corner office, indicating that I was the boss, and I could tell it was over a multi-faceted, umbrella organization. My desk was neat and I was standing beside this beautiful deep mahogany or cherry wood desk. I was in a tailored pantsuit, and I was slim and trim. I was the epitome of discipline in that vision. As I came out of the vision, I looked at the chaos that was around me with stacks of unorganized papers everywhere and overweight then I looked up as if looking to God and said, "Whatever you have to do to get me from here to there…DO IT!" I keep that vision before me, especially now since I've been on my journey. I am striving to get to that version of myself. I want to be in that position and in that body, so I keep a mental image of it.

I've also created a vision board for this journey (I've included a picture of it on the next page). Since I've never been to the place I'm trying to go in my adult life, I don't have a final picture, but I have a picture that is a size 12 that has always been an inspiration to me. I have included it along with the picture of where I was when I started this journey. I have my size-12-motivation picture and my frame with a "Coming Soon" sign on it for where I will be. I also have some motivational quotes and some pictures of some outfits I want to wear when I get there.

Keeping mental and visual images before you will help you resist temptation when it comes, and push you to work out on those days when you don't feel like it. Remember, every action and decision you make will get you closer to or farther away from your goals, so what choice will you make?

I'd like you to take a moment and write down your Defining Moment. What is your reason for starting this journey?

____

____

____

____

____

____

____

____

____

____

____

____

Vision Board

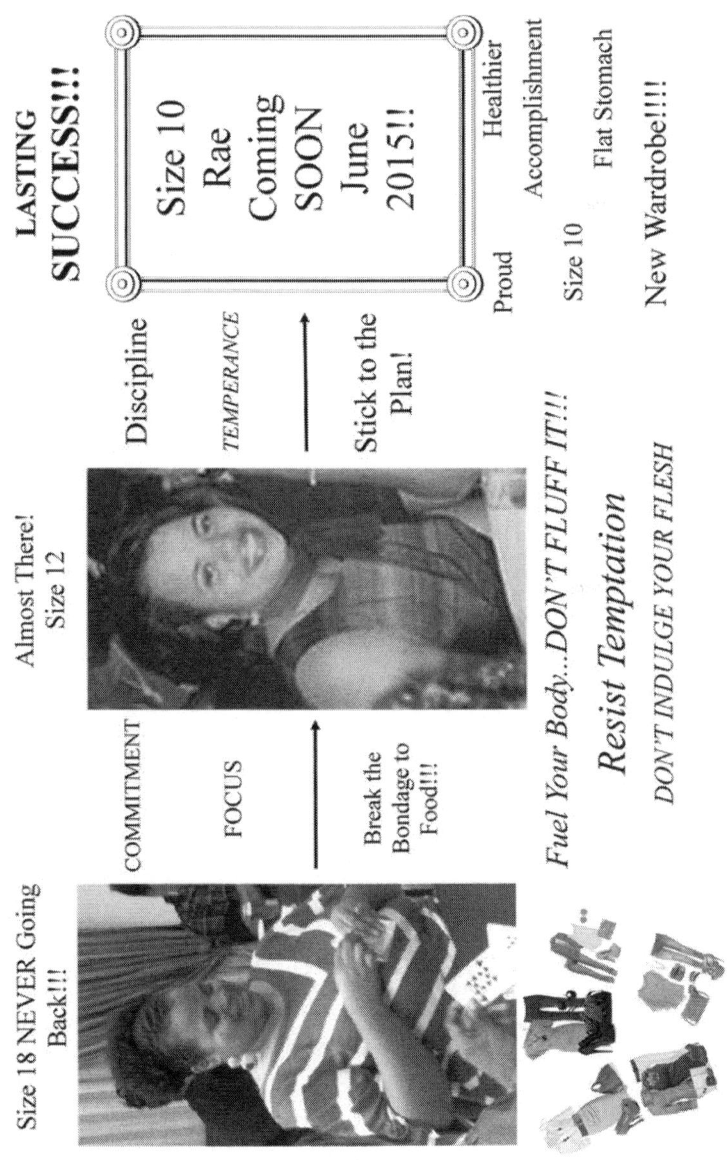

Chapter Two
Key #2: Make a Plan

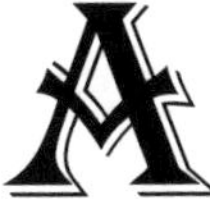 plan is defined as a scheme or method of acting, doing, proceeding, making, etc. developed in advance.

What is your plan of action? You must have a plan or else you WILL fail. So, what will you do for exercise? How will you modify your eating? What will your water intake be? Will you take supplements, if so, which ones?

Why does an architect have to create plans for a building before it gets built? So that everyone working on the building knows what they are supposed to be doing, and what the end result needs to look like. There is no guesswork, everyone knows exactly what he or she needs to be doing and all they have to do is follow the plan. This alleviates confusion, accidents, and failure.

A plan is a detailed roadmap that helps you get to where you are going and allows all your members to prepare the journey in which you are about to embark upon. It tells you what steps to take to get to your desired destination. Without a plan, how will you know if you're on track and will arrive on time? How will you know that you have not deviated from the course onto a path of disappointment?

What Plan Works for You?

There are TONS of weight-loss options available, but you must decide which one will work best for you. I personally think deprivation is a poor choice. We must view this as a lifestyle change, not a diet. A diet is temporary, but what we are doing is changing our lifestyle; the way we eat, when we eat, what we eat, when we exercise, what exercise we do, etc. This has to be something that you will be able to implement in your life.

Be realistic! If you love carbs, but you go on a diet that does not allow you to have carbs the one time you sneak and have carbs, you will undo all that you've done because you haven't had them. You will overindulge and could possibly end up worse off than when you started. Not to mention we do need some carbohydrates because they provide fuel to our bodies. The key is moderation, not long periods of deprivation. When we deprive ourselves, then all we think about is all the wonderful things we're going to eat when we get off this "diet". Well, this is what causes us to end up gaining back more weight than what we lost.

Find a plan that works for you. Personally, the Shred Diet worked wonderfully for me. It allowed me to eat several small meals per day, along with some snacks in between, so my body didn't feel deprived and caused me to want to overindulge later on. This is a personal choice. You have to find what works best for you and will allow you to stick to the plan that you can possibly incorporate into your new lifestyle.

Also, you must determine your exercise plan. You absolutely need to do some sort of calorie burning exercises: riding a bike in your neighborhood or a stationary bike, walking in your neighborhood or on a treadmill, or using other equipment like an elliptical machine. Maybe you enjoy group classes like Zumba, Step, aerobics, Piloxing, MixxedFit, line dancing class, swimming, water aerobics, workout to videos at home, or calisthenics. Anything, or a combination of these things, would be great to get you started. You just need to get active and get that heart pumping! Just make sure it's something that you will enjoy doing. It is crucial as you are just getting started or restarting an exercise routine that you do something that you will enjoy and have fun doing. If it feels too much like a workout right at the beginning, you may be tempted to stop because it's too hard and not fun.

Personally, when I started back, I had to do what was

enjoyable. I enjoyed walking in my neighborhood and it gave me a sense of accomplishment when I would push myself to go farther and farther. When I started going to the gym, I needed classes that were fun. The hard stuff was not my cup of tea, but coming to Zumba to dance, smile, and have fun was exactly what I needed. Zumba is not for everyone, and I could not begin to understand those folks that enjoyed the cycling (spinning) class. I tried it a couple of times, and I had absolutely NO fun! I hated it the entire time and could not wait to get out of the class. As a matter-of-fact, the first time I took the starter class, I left early! It was 15 minutes into it and my daughter had decided to join me. I looked over at her and asked, "Are you ready to leave?" and she said, "YES!" so we slipped out early.

As time went on, I came to the point where I began to feel stronger and more confident. I started branching out to trying new things. I first introduced myself to an abs (abdominals) class, which I was terribly afraid to try for fear of not being able to do it. Then I branched out to a Piloxing class, which fuses boxing with Pilate's movements, which was intense. I always joked with my instructor that I had a "Love-Hate" relationship with Piloxing, but I never stopped showing up. Being able to take that class gave me the confidence to want to try Boot Camp, which is a military style, intense workout. Along the way, I began to incorporate weight training into my routine. The last hurdle for me to cross was cycling. I incurred an injury at one point, a torn tendon in my ankle, and I had to modify my exercise routines. I couldn't do Zumba for 3 months. Well, I started picking up weight due to a significant decrease in my normal work out routine. My Boot Camp instructor encouraged me to give Cycling a try. She said it was a great, effective workout and the pain from the seat would be gone in a week. Well, I tried it and actually began to like it (since it was the only high-intensity work out I could do). Now, I incorporate it into my weekly routine.

Now for those of you that are hard-core and really like to go "all in" on your workouts, you can go for it. I am really speaking to those that are similar to me. In the past, I had a tendency to start intense, and then lose my momentum burning out in a period of about six months or sooner. So, this time, I recognized my weakness, and decided to try to enjoy my workout until I got to the point where working out became a regular part of my life and a priority to me. So, if you're like me, start with having fun, the WORK out will come later!

Setting Your Goals

Many times, when we set a goal for our weight-loss, we set a large number and say we want to lose that in a short amount of time. Well, unless you're doing some unhealthy manner of losing weight, that goal is unreasonable.

First off, many doctors and health experts recommend that you only lose one to two pounds per week. When we first start our program, we are going to most likely lose larger numbers than that because we move from doing nothing to actively working towards our goal weight. The sudden activity will cause us to lose more in the beginning. But, we will have to keep steadily working at it and "bump it up" as we progress on our journey in order to continue our weight-loss.

When setting your goals, don't be anxious. You didn't gain the weight overnight; it will take time for all that you want to lose to come off. There is a saying that really freed me when I learned it. "How do you eat an elephant? One bite at a time." Saying, I want to lose 80 pounds can be an overwhelming thought when you initially say it, but saying, "I want to lose six pounds per month for the next 12 months sounds a lot more attainable.

Break your goal weight down into manageable "mini-monthly goals". Shoot for five pounds per month and just keep striving toward that goal. You'd be surprised at how large of a role your mindset plays in your weight-loss success.

Do Your Research

Find out how many glasses of water you need to drink, what supplements will aid you in your process, what the benefits of lemon water, and other suggestions are. Become active in your weight-loss journey instead of blindly doing what the plan says. When you understand why they are saying these things are beneficial, it will help you not to deviate from the plan as much.

Planning Is Key

While on your particular plan, you have to prepare ahead of time. You don't want to wait until it's time to eat to figure out what you're going to eat. In that moment of hunger, you are more susceptible to impulse eating because you just want to satisfy that hunger pang. Plan your meals in advance: a day, even a week in advance. Go shopping; get the items that you will need for your meals and snacks. Organization is going to be crucial to your success. You definitely want to set yourself up for success, so make sure that you have healthy snacking options within reach instead of unhealthy, high calorie/fat options. Make a schedule for your eating so that you are able to eat according to the plan instead of according to pang! My 30 Day Exercise & Nutrition Plan is a great companion to this book to help you with this task.

Stick to the Plan!

Do everything within your power to stick to your plan.

You will be challenged like never before in this, but you MUST do it! You CAN do it! With your mind made up, you can do ANYTHING!!! If you have a craving for something that is not on your meal plan, you have to get that thought out of your mind as quickly as possible. The trouble comes when we entertain the thought. There is a scripture in the bible, Matthew 5:28, that tells us that if a man looks at a woman and lusts after her in his heart then he has already committed adultery. James 1:14 says that "But every man is tempted, when he is drawn away of his own lust and enticed". Let me tie these two scriptures together in relation to our discussion concerning our weight-loss journey.

First, a question: What happens in that moment that the man lusts after her? What has happened is that he has allowed a thought that is a part of his lust or desire to occupy his mind, so he has entertained that thought. We cannot be tempted with anything that is not appealing to us. If it doesn't appeal to me, it can't entice me. However, if it is something that deep down I desire, or struggle with, then it has the potential to entice me. Back to our scenario of our man, the thought was introduced in his mind; however, he didn't have to accept the thought. He could have immediately rejected it, but because it was a desire or longing, he allowed it to linger and he entertains the idea and plays out the entire experience in his mind-psychologically experiencing the pleasure of it. What has he done? He has set himself up for a fall!

It's the same way with our eating. If a thought of eating something not on our plan is introduced to us, we have to immediately reject it. We cannot allow ourselves to entertain that thought. If we imagine how it will taste or feel in our mouths with the explosion of flavors we will experience, we have already set ourselves up to fail! This is a struggle that I have. I LOVE peanut M&M's. I ate bags and bags of them when I was breast-feeding my (now 11-

year-old) daughter as a baby. I am STILL working off the pounds I gained during that time. When the thought of indulging in some of them is introduced to me and I don't immediately arrest the thought and reject it, I will play the scenario out of how I would place the wonderful piece of chocolate and peanut delicately wrapped in a thin crunchy candy shell to the side of my tongue for a few seconds, allowing it to melt, and just as the coating begins to break down, I would crunch through it, experiencing the explosion of chocolate and reach the ultimate goal of that crunchy peanut hidden beneath. Now…if I just made you crave peanut M&M's, I apologize…but DON'T DO IT!!!! You don't have to receive that thought; you can REJECT IT!

If we don't capture and immediately reject those thoughts, we will give in to them. Then we, like moths to the flame, will be blindly driven to move heaven and earth if we have to in order to fulfill this desire. There have been times I've gotten in my car and gone to the store to fulfill a craving that I had! The craving was so strong because I allowed it to hang in my mind that I had to entertain it. If I entertain it, just as that scripture in Matthew says, I will indulge, and so will you!

If You Fall

There is an expression that says, "The best laid plans of mice and men oft go astray." That means that things often go wrong even after you have carefully planned what you are going to do. Let's face it; there are times when we will deviate from our plan. Some people like to factor in "cheat days" into their regimen in order to allow their desire to be appeased in an effort to stay on track the rest of the week; if that's you and it works for you, then great. I personally cannot do that. Now, does that mean I always stick to the plan? Nope, I sure do not! I deviate from time-to-time;

probably more times than I'd care to admit.

So, what do you do if you fall? Do you give the whole idea of losing weight up? No, you get back up, dust yourself off, acknowledge that you messed up and analyze what caused you to mess up. How did you not make it? What was going on at that moment? How did you become vulnerable? Which one of your guards was down that you missed and caused you to be open to attack? Yes, when you are bombarded with thoughts that are contrary to your plan, you are under attack! Your appetite wants to take you back to where you've come from, but you have to recognize your vulnerability and close up that area of your wall. Are you an emotional eater? Do you eat when you're sad, stressed, bored, etc.? This is your vulnerability. Instead of eating something that is not on your plan or at an unscheduled time according to your plan, do something else; go for a walk, drink some water. Research and find out why you're craving what and when you're craving it.

According to Dr. Colleen Huber, a Naturopathic Medical Doctor, she states that, "cravings are actually the manifestation of a mild malnutrition" (http://natureworks best.com/naturopathy-works/food-cravings/). Sometimes, your body will crave nutrients that you are deficient in and it will manifest in a way that you are familiar with. For example, you may crave carbs or bread. Well, that may be because your body is depleted in its stores of the mineral selenium, which is found in flour. So, instead of white bread, choose wholegrain bread or even Brazil nuts to satisfy that craving. If you crave chips or salty foods, it may be a sign of adrenal fatigue (related to constant stress), so choose air-popped popcorn or nuts instead. Also, be sure to get enough sleep. If you're craving meat, your body may need more protein, so be sure to increase your protein intake."[1]

I recognize that there are certain places that I go to that trigger a craving. For instance, when I go to the mall near our house, I always crave Chinese food and cookies from Mrs. Fields. That's because we ate that when we went to the mall once, and every time I go back, I want it. This happens with me often. If I've experienced a food item that was enjoyable or pleasurable, at or near a place, my appetite will want to recreate the experience and triggers a craving when I am in that environment. That's because there are chemical releases that occur when we are eating, and one of those is *dopamine*. There is an almost "euphoric" experience that occurs if it was enjoyable or connected with a pleasurable experience. This is the same chemical release during a romantic sexual encounter (which makes you stay longer in something than you should, but that's another book for another day), as well as the experience that keeps people addicted to drugs. They keep trying to recreate that "high". So, back to weight-loss, if we eat something at a place, or if we have a pleasurable experience at a place, it will release dopamine. Well, when we think about, get to, or near the trigger location again, it will cause us to crave that experience again. You have to understand the trigger and if you are simply trying to have a pleasurable experience related to food, recognize what is going on and realize it's just your body trying to get an emotional "high". Reject the thought and find something else that makes you happy and keep moving!

---

[1] Atkinson, L. (2010, June 14). Curb those cravings! Knowing why you get that insatiable urge for a bar of chocolate is the first step to beating it. *The Daily Mail*. Retrieved from http://dailymail.co.uk/femail/ article-1286393/Curb-cravings-knowing-insatiable-urge-bar-chocolate-step-beating-it.html

If You Fail to Plan, You Plan to Fail

Devise your plan. It helps you to be focused and prepared for the drastic changes that you're about to make in your life. Preparation is crucial to success as it enables you to feel more in control and more empowered, helping to ensure your success.

There are a plethora of eating plans out there: Weight Watchers, NutriSystem, Shred Diet, Atkins Diet, Green smoothie (a 10-day plan to jump start your weight-loss), and so on and so forth. You just have to look at the ones that are right for you, understand it, make your food purchase preparations, start it, and STICK TO THE PLAN!

What Is Your Plan?

What eating regimen will you employ to lose weight and what will it entail?

___

___

___

___

___

___

___

___

___

___

___

___

What will your exercise regimen consist of? (i.e. what type of cardio, what type of strength training, how often will you go, and for how long?)

____

____

____

____

____

____

____

____

____

____

____

What places do you go to that trigger an eating response in you, and what type of response is it? (What foods do you crave when you go there?)

____

____

____

____

____

____

____

____

What will your response be when a craving comes up that is contrary to your plan?

What will you do to stay motivated on those days when you don't feel like sticking to your workout regimen?

Chapter Three
Key #3: Accountability

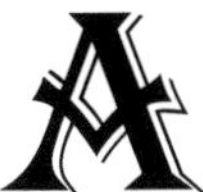ccountability is defined as: Liable to account for one's actions; liable to be called to account; answerable to someone else.

If you are going to be successful on this journey, a crucial key is that you are going to have to be accountable to someone else. You will have to find yourself an accountability partner or "Buddy" as we call it in the Fitness Finesse with Rae Accountability Group. Having to account for your actions and eating habits will help you stay on task. As you make decisions about whether or not you will work out or what you will eat, you will have the accountability buddy in the back of your mind. In our Accountability Group we have a challenge that we've adopted called "The 8-Month Challenge". These individuals have set a goal that they will work towards over an 8-month period running from October to June. So we take the fall, winter, and spring to work towards our goal so that we will be ready for the summer. These "Buddy Teams" have developed names for their teams and are holding each other accountable to their exercise and eating regimens. Some workout together, most do not, but they report or post pictures of their meal choices and exercise activities for each day. This has been extremely motivational and has inspired many to eat better, workout more, drink water, and take the necessary steps to reaching their goals. The "team" mindset helps them to push harder and stick to their plan because they subconsciously feel that if they don't, they are letting their teammates down. This has been an extremely successful strategy to help these individuals jump-start their weight-loss journey. At the time of this writing, we have one person that has lost 40 pounds and another that has lost 24 as a result of this group. Others are inspired by the pictures and posts that their fellow group members are posting that it has motivated them to step up their activity in their work outs.

For me accountability was something that I shied away from. When I first started my journey, I decided that this time I wouldn't tell anyone that I had started yet another weight-loss journey. See, I've started and stopped so many diets in my lifetime, and when I started this one, I had just started one the year before and stopped yet again. I lost some weight and was doing good until I fell off and ended up gaining back more than what I'd lost, leaving me at my 247 pounds. I was afraid to tell anyone I was starting again because, "What if I stopped again?" However, I was more afraid to stop this time because I might cross that 250-pound mark, and I was afraid that I would balloon up to 300 pounds if I stopped this time. So I started my journey, and three weeks into it was my birthday. My mom wanted to take me shopping for my birthday, so that day I got up and got dressed. I was feeling kind of cute, so I asked my husband to take my picture. Well, he did, and just before I was about to leave, he put my "before" picture and the picture he had just taken side by side and he said, "Bae…you HAVE to see this!" I said, "See what?" He showed me the pictures and I was blown away. There was a TREMENDOUS and noticeable difference between Week 1 and Week 3. I was excited and encouraged as I prepared to go looking for new clothes. While I was at the store I picked out a "little black dress"—because every woman needs to have one of those in her closet—and I was debating on the size. Excited about my three-week victory, I hesitantly told my mom that I wasn't sure which one I should get because I had just started a new diet and I wanted to buy for my future weight. I was hesitant to tell her because she knew all the weight battles I've had throughout my life and has seen me start and stop many diets. My telling her would then make me accountable to her for another one, and I wasn't quite ready to tell anyone. I wanted to wait until my six weeks was over and then people would see what I had accomplished. However, I didn't want to waste her money, so I told her what I was doing. Because she knew my track record, when I told her, she gave me this look of, "yeah right, you know how this is going to end", but she said, "OK, try on the 14".

When I got in the dressing room, I tried on several of the outfits and she could tell I had lost some weight, however when I got to the "little black dress", she said, "Wow! You *have* lost weight! What are you doing?" I then told her about the Shred Diet. The next day, I sent her the before and after picture my husband took and she was blown away. She emailed it to her co-workers, printed it out, and showed it to my aunts and uncles and everyone was asking, "What is she doing? I need to do that!" So many of them purchased and began the Shred Diet after that. I wasn't ready for her to do that—I didn't want all those eyes on me! What if I couldn't hold out? What if I failed-again? I was hesitant about all this attention, and yet at the same time, I really couldn't believe the results I had gotten. It was a drastic difference in such a short amount of time. So I posted the pictures on Facebook. My page EXPLODED! I had about 125 likes in less than a day and about 95 comments from people asking me what I was doing. It even caught the attention of the creator of the diet, Dr. Ian Smith. He asked me to send him my before and after picture for consideration for his commercial. I didn't get picked, but something was happening. All this attention—all these eyes on my journey—it did something to me. It pushed me to go farther. It was driving me to keep it up, to not quit and to make it happen. I felt as if all these people were counting on me to do it so that they could know that they could do it too. It's hard to explain the feelings I was having, but I felt as though my weight loss journey became my responsibility to others. In my mind, I felt that I *had* to succeed this time, because so many people were depending on me to do it. There were naysayers along the way, people that said, "Yeah, I know someone that started it and lost weight, but they ended up gaining it back". Instead of discouraging me, that actually fueled my motivation even more to prove that no matter what other people's experiences were, *I* was going to succeed.

I was terrified at the beginning, but now I am so grateful that my mother made me accountable. She pushed me into an aspect of my destiny that I didn't even see coming. Not in A MILLION years did I EVER think I would be a Fitness Advocate. I admired people that were athletes and secretly wished that I had been athletically inclined. I felt that they were programmed with the ability to discipline themselves and were wired to work out vigorously and not despise it. I wished I had been born with that drive, ambition, and enjoyment of self-torture that I viewed exercise to be. Now here I am today—a year and a half later—and I LOVE to work out! Recently, I even had a fitness instructor tell me that I inspired her! She had gotten discouraged in her fitness journey, but seeing my posts of my work outs motivated and inspired her to get back in the game. I am developing more and more discipline and taking more control over my body. I am at the gym five to seven days a week, twice a day sometimes most times. I absolutely love getting my work out in and making it a part of my day. I look at myself now and say, "Who is this person?" I am a COMPLETELY different person than who I used to be and I LOVE it! Where I am today, I know beyond a shadow of a doubt, that I would not be here without my mother and her actions of making me accountable for what I had committed to doing for myself.

That being said, accountability only works if you *make* yourself accountable to another person or to other people. If you try to hold back, hide, or give yourself an "out" just in case you don't make it, then you will not make it! You will excuse yourself and agree with yourself when you don't feel like working out or when you don't want to deny yourself the bowl of butter pecan ice cream. However, if you make yourself accountable to someone, every decision you make will run through your mental filter of accountability. It will change the food and exercise decisions you make. It will push you to work out when you don't feel like it. When you have to report your weight or progress, you will want to make sure you have made progress because there are other people counting on you. No one can want it for you, you have to want it for yourself and push yourself beyond your comfort zone and limitations in order to reach your goals. Having a person or group of people that you have to answer to helps to push you to do what it takes to make those goals possible.

Is Having an Accountability Network Really That Important?

Well, let's look at the statistics from an online article in the NEA Member Benefits page: (www.m.neamb.com/ shopping-discounts/buddy-weight-loss-htm)

- The Journal of American Medical Association published a study in which more than 400 overweight and obese women participating in the Jenny Craig Program (weekly one-on-one consultations, personalized nutrition, and activity plans) achieved an average weight-loss of 10% of their body weight after one year and nearly 8% at the two year mark, compared with self-dieters who lost 2% of their body weight.
- Researchers at the University of Pennsylvania compared solo participants to those who work out with a few friends and found that:

  - Those who had buddies were more likely to stick with the programs 95% vs. 24%
  - Those who had buddies maintained their loss 66% vs. 24%
- Also:
  - Jim White, R.D. spokesperson for the American Dietetic Association stated the following:
    - "Group weight-loss challenges are a great source of motivation and provide an opportunity for participants to vent to one another, release frustrations, share tips, and motivational stories to promote success"
    - The article goes on to state that seeing your team members succeed may inspire you to work harder.
    - Lastly, the article states that when it comes to participating in an exercise plan, there's a 60% dropout rate within six months and by partnering with a trainer or another gym member you'll increase your odds of success.

So, based upon those numbers and personal experience, I would say that having an Accountability Buddy is certainly a way to ensure success for your weight-loss goals.

Some Tips for Choosing an Accountability Buddy

Groups:

- If there are groups available, check those out. You may have a group at work or church or some other organization you belong to that may be on a weight-loss journey, ask around. If not, why not start one yourself? If you know of a group of individuals that are ready to get started on a weight-loss journey, get them together and get going! If that's not your cup of tea, you can always look online for a virtual accountability group, like Fitness Finesse w/Rae. You are always welcome to join our Accountability Group. We provide motivation, inspiration, support, encouragement, and friendly competition as we strive to reach our weight-loss goals.

Like-Minded Individuals

- Try to find individuals that are already on a fitness plan, or are seriously motivated to start one. (There can be a challenge that arises when someone is not fully committed to making the changes and doing the work that is necessary when committing to a weight-loss journey.) Connecting with people that are serious and focused on achieving goals is crucial, especially if you don't have a solid support system at home that you can look to. If you have a fitness center membership, it may help to look there first. If there is someone that you regularly see at the same classes or gym time as you, befriend them to see if they may be willing to be your accountability or workout buddy and schedule workout times that you all can do together.

Connect with People You Actually Like

- This is common sense, but it still may need to be stated. Find someone that has a personality that you can get along with well. Someone that will challenge you, but support you at the same time and even understand the struggles you are having and relate to them, but will also help you get over obstacles and push through them to help you put forth your best effort.

Tips for a Successful Buddy or Team Experience

- Set goals for your team. What is your yearly, monthly, and weekly goal? Will you drink 6-8 glasses of water a day? Will you incorporate more types of new exercises into your work out week (i.e. squats, push ups, sit ups, etc.)? As a group, set your goals and work toward those goals either together or individually with a report to the team being required.

- Stay connected to your team members. Get their phone numbers, emails, and social media information so that you can stay connected to them. You will need to keep in contact daily, even several times a day to ensure that everyone is on track with the goals.

If you have tried unsuccessfully to stick to a weight-loss plan in the past or lost weight but were unable to maintain the loss, what do you think was the reason you were unsuccessful?

____

____

____

____

____

____

____

____

____

____

____

Do you feel that you could make yourself accountable to someone this time around? Why or Why not?

____

____

Who do you think you could be held accountable to? (Individual or Group)

Chapter Four
Key #4: Support System

The definition of "support" is: To hold in position so as to keep from falling, sinking, or slipping; to keep from weakening or failing; to strengthen.

Having a support system is absolutely critical in your weight-loss journey. No man is an island unto himself, meaning that no one is absolutely self-sufficient. We all need others in our lives to help us in some way, form, or fashion. This could not be a more true statement as it relates to a successful weight-loss journey. Leading up to my journey in February 2013, I was at a place where I had trained myself to eat without restraint for so long, that I could not muster the mindset to do it on my own. I had become so frustrated with myself that I had basically given up. I had resolved that it was my lot in life to be a "Big Girl", even though deep down inside there was a smaller version of myself that I knew was screaming to come out—the more disciplined one that I saw in my vision. Remember that I told you that my husband is a snacker. He would keep a stash of cakes, cookies, chips, and candy by his side of the bed. For the most part, I would not buy these types of things because I knew that I would eat them, and I was attempting to practice restraint by not purchasing them. Not to say I don't snack. My logic was if I don't buy it, there's less temptation to eat it. However, when he would snack, the thoughts of the taste of those snacks would flood my mind, and I would give in to temptation. We would sit in the bed and munch and snack on those delectable, detrimental goodies while watching television.

Now, I will say that his snacking has slacked off tremendously, not to say he doesn't enjoy an occasional snack, but now he chooses healthier options like fruits or granola bars. He has actually lost 60 pounds since February

2013, and the last few pounds he did by not snacking. I've never seen anyone drop weight so quickly by not snacking! I'm so jealous!

For me, it was easier to lose weight when he was not snacking. The temptation was removed because it was not easily accessible. Additionally, when we both decided to start the Shred Diet together, it helped that we were on the same track, eating the same foods. It's hard when you have one person eating healthy, and the other eating everything else. This was a tremendous help to my weight-loss efforts. Additionally, it helped when he wanted to go to the gym to workout. On days when I wasn't feeling it, he would push me and vice versa. We were each other's accountability and support.

Not only that, but he was my biggest cheerleader. He would encourage me to go to the gym and participate in the classes. I am fortunate because I've met ladies at the gym who said that their husband's have complained about all the time they spend at the gym, but that was not my case. My husband was very supportive of my rigorous workout routine. There were days when I would be there for two-and-half to three hours taking various classes. He never complained. He would come with me some days, and others he would have to stay home because he had limited mobility due to a knee injury. Either way, he encouraged me to keep pressing, especially as he saw me making significant progress. He knew that this was important to me, he knew the goal that we were on, and he reaped the benefits of a slimmer, healthier wife as well!

Support of Loved Ones is Crucial

Having the support of your loved ones and those you live with is crucial to your success. Share with them your desire to lose weight and your reasons for it. Ask them to workout with you, but if they're not ready, ask them to at least support you by not triggering your weaknesses. I chuckle as I write this because there was one time when my husband hid a bag of M & M's in his car in order to not tempt me with them! He didn't bring them into the house because he knew they were my kryptonite!

Meal planning can also be a challenge when you are the only one on a weight loss journey. Having to prepare high-calorie, rich foods for your family while having to eat bean sprouts can be a serious challenge for any one. But, developing a healthier way of cooking is good for your whole family. That's why we must look at this as a lifestyle change, not a diet. A Diet says, "This is temporary and I only have to endure this for a little while". A lifestyle change is changing the status quo for my household and me.

Many of the issues with food and our association with it come from our childhood. If we are raising children, it is our responsibility to teach them healthy eating and nutrition habits while they are young. It will probably have to be a slow introduction; however, kids have an amazing ability to adapt to change—even if they don't like it initially. In many of the school systems, they are adopting healthier menus, removing bad snacks out of vending machines, and giving them healthy eating education. We should take advantage of that and introduce these healthier options into our homes as well as what they are learning. We don't want to pass diabetes, hypertension, and other weight-related issues on to our children. Nor do we want to lose our spouses to these diseases. Eating healthier is good for the whole family, so make it a point to bring everyone on to the weight-loss journey just by making healthier meals and providing snacks with better nutritional value. You may not be able to change the whole structure that your house has been built on because your loved ones may still want their usual snacks to some degree, but it is in these moments where your self-restraint will need to kick in.

Develop a Support System with other Like-minded Individuals

When we first rejoined the YMCA, I started attending Zumba classes. I stayed in the back and kept to myself. I didn't know anyone and just came and went without connecting with other people. As time went on, I continued to go and started seeing the same people showing up for the same classes. I started to get to know them and connect with them. After a short while, I would look them up on Facebook and would request to be their friend. As they would post about their weight-loss journey, I began to get inspired in mine. There would be days when I didn't feel like working out, but I would log onto Facebook and see one of them post about being excited to go workout, and it would inspire me. When I wanted to sit on the couch and do nothing, it made me want to get up and get moving. I began to get excited about going to class, and there was an amazing energy that would be in the class because we were all on the same mission and same goal. We would feed off of each other's energy and motivation and it would push us to greater limits beyond our comfort zone. It has created a real bond because it developed a "we're all in this together" mentality. It was a unified goal that we were all working towards and we were doing it together.

Not only that, but our instructors subconsciously became our "fearless leaders", guiding us to victory in the war against the bulge. They would push us and challenge us to go beyond where we had ever been before. Personally, I went kicking and screaming, but because I was accountable to them, I trusted them to take me to new heights so that I could reach places I had never been. I wanted to make them proud. I was willing to and had let myself down many times when I was the only person I was accountable to; but when it came to them, these people that I felt believed in me and my ability to do it, I pushed myself to do things I never thought were possible.

All of these people were my rock and the reasons I have been as successful this time around. I have developed a new mindset toward health and fitness, and it is because of the support and accountability that I've had this time around on my journey. I tried many times, but I COULD NOT do it by myself. I absolutely must have a support system to help me achieve my goals. Without this support system of workout buddies, loved ones, and amazing instructors who won't let me quit and won't let me say "I can't", I would not be where I am today. There is one person that I am extremely grateful to, and that is Dr. Ian Smith. His program came along at just the time I needed it. I know that the events in my life that led up to me looking for eating plans were divinely orchestrated. I am just grateful that Dr. Smith was diligent to write it. He made a statement when promoting his book that he was done writing weight-loss books that he had said all he had to say about them. Well, I'm eternally grateful that he took one more time to write a book that would help people. It has truly changed my life and the course of it. It is because of him that I am even writing this book today, and have created a Health & Wellness Ministry that is helping people overcome their challenges and hindrances to losing weight. By him walking in his purpose, it has allowed me to walk in mine, and I am eternally grateful!

You must develop a support system. Get your spouse, grab a loved one or friend, or find a gym buddy. Someone that can motivate, push, encourage, challenge, strengthen, and support you through this process. No man is an island unto himself; we all need someone to help us through the various facets of life. Having a solid support system in your weight loss efforts will help ensure you reach your goals. I've shown you the many layers of support I've had in my journey. Now you must develop yours.

Questions…

Who will my support system be?

If I don't have one, where can I find one?

What will I need from my support system?

Chapter Five
Key #5: Take an Introspective Look

Temptation was always the challenge for me in losing weight over the years. I would get the mindset, set my plan, and get started. I would be doing well for a while and then I would begin to have moments of weakness. Instead of resisting those thoughts, I would give in, and most times I wasn't even hungry; I just wanted to eat. This has been one of my biggest challenges in my life. I wouldn't necessarily be hungry instead I would just want to eat. This was so distressing to me because many times, I could not tell if I was truly hungry, or just driven by a desire to eat. Many times I wasn't fulfilling a natural need to eat, but I was fueling a desire to eat. I felt like a slave to food and more so my appetite.

As I earnestly prayed and sought God about this, I received an answer, which was that my eating was my indulgence. It was the one place in my life that I had no restraint and my body showed the fruit of that lack of restraint. My justification was, "Well, we have to eat! That's why food was put here, we need food to live". It was not until years later that I would come to understand that food has been given to us as fuel for our bodies, but we often use it to fluff our bodies instead. All food is not good food, meaning that it is not beneficial for us. There is no nutritional value in certain foods or the way certain foods are prepared. We have to be honest with ourselves and really take inventory of the foods we enjoy eating to see if we are using food for its intended purpose, or to fulfill our guilty pleasures.

After a workshop I presented on this subject recently, I had an individual come up to me and tell me I could use her story. She said that she too was praying about her weight issue, and she received an answer that stated she was killing herself with her mouth. The bad eating choices she was making were actually causing her to slowly kill herself. How so? Health conditions brought on by being overweight, such as diabetes, heart disease, stroke, high blood pressure, some cancers, sleep apnea, and others, are serious health conditions that could eventually take your life.

When we initially started our Accountability Group, we had 68 women and no men. Women continued to see our promotions and wanted to do something about their weight, but men would simply blow it off. I want to share a heartfelt plea that my husband shared in an attempt to get more men to get serious about their health and connect with our Accountability Group so that they could begin to get healthy as well:

> *"I first had a talk with God, who reminded me that our body is the temple that houses the Holy Spirit, and this temple needed to be renovated...That there are too many who profess to be His, that are suffering in a temple on the verge of being condemned...that how can we be witnesses to a body of people, when we are a poor example of temperance... that we are committing physical suicide, because of our inability to bring our flesh under subjection. My wife and I made a vow to each other and God, that we were committed to lose the weight by exercise and proper diet, that snacks would be in smaller quantity, add more fiber, and drink more water. It just came down to the fact that I did not want to die by my own hand. You see diabetes, hypertension, strokes, and heart attacks happen mostly because of us... And the funny thing is once I lost the first 20 pounds, I no longer needed the CPAT*

machine (for sleep apnea), when I got to 229 pounds, my blood sugar went back to normal levels... Men, we as the head of our households need to do the same, getting our temples in shape. I don't know about you, but I refuse to die by something that I can control."

I understand that many of us have many different reasons for our weight struggles, but we must be willing to take an honest, open look at ourselves in the mirror within to see what is really going on. Whether we overeat, under eat, have a slow metabolism, are "big-boned", etc., there is an issue going on that we have to be willing to come face-to-face with. Why do we have the behavior that has led to our weight gain? Why do we not want to workout? Why don't we eat enough or why do we eat too much? I guarantee there is a deeper issue at the root of all of our weight issues that if unaddressed will continue to hinder our efforts. Once we see it, we have to muster up the drive and determination to deal with it and do what is necessary to correct it at all cost, because our lives depend on it.

Questions...

Take some time and give some thought and prayer to your reasons for your eating habits.

Do you eat too often? Too much? Not enough? When not hungry? Take some time and do some soul-searching to find out, why. Why are you eating this way? As you begin to process how you eat, what you eat, and why you eat the way you do, you will come to discover some things about yourself that you may not have known or recognized before. (This may take some time to discover the answer, but allow it to marinate in your mind and spirit and you will hear the answer come to you.) Write your discoveries here:

____

Now, armed with this revelation, what is your plan for addressing what you've learned? What are you going to do with this knowledge? You must have a plan for overcoming this issue so that it is gone once and for all and so that it doesn't hinder you any longer. Write your plan here:

Chapter Six
Key #6: Back to Mindset

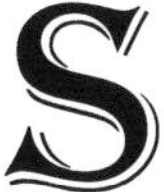tarting and continuing this journey starts and ends with your mindset. You will constantly have to renew your mind to this lifestyle change.

Remember Why You Started

Inevitably, there are going to be times when you just are not "feeling it". Days will come when you don't want to work out; you may have had a hard day at work, a sleepless night, you may be stressed or weary. There are days when you don't want to eat healthy, when you will just want to indulge and enjoy some junk food. There will be days when you're too tired to cook or prepare meals in advance.

However, it is in these times that you have to go back and remember why you started this journey in the first place. Go back and look at your defining moment. What was your reason for starting? Is that reason still the same? Then allow it to push you back into the mindset you need to get back on the plan. Look at your vision board. Which path are your efforts supposed to steer you on? What are you working towards? Are you on track or are you veering off course? Every decision you make – whether or not to workout, whether or not to indulge, whether or not to prepare and plan – will affect your success. Depending upon the decision you make, will get you closer to or farther away from your goals. You have to stay focused on your goals and stay motivated.

There are days when I don't have the motivation that I need, but then I remember where I came from and how I don't EVER want to go back there again, and it causes me to press on. I didn't have physical health conditions, but mentally I had tremendous self-esteem and self-worth issues. I didn't feel good about myself because I felt weak and undisciplined, and that upset me because one of the Fruits of the Spirit is "Temperance," which means self-discipline. My body screamed a lack of discipline and I felt that was bringing shame to God. I tried to be satisfied being a "Big Girl," but it didn't look good on me. I didn't wear weight well at all! My ankles were fat and looked swollen, my thighs and legs looked like one long limb; I had zero definition and my knees had all but disappeared. I had a double chin and a really fat face. I even looked older. I didn't realize I was looking older until I started losing weight and started looking younger. I could not believe what the weight was doing to my physical appearance and mental image of myself. Weight was not my friend at all! It was having all kinds of negative effects on my life.

Maybe your goal is to get to a certain dress size, get off medication, attend an event, get healthy for your family, or whatever! Keep that goal in mind. In those moments when you want to cheat or give up all together – REMEMBER WHY YOU STARTED! If that condition has not changed, then you still need to stay committed to this journey. You may need to call on your Accountability Buddies in an Emergency 911 situation, and simply thinking about your commitment to them is not enough to do it! That's what they're there for.

Stay Committed

One of the best ways to stay committed to your weight loss journey is to stay connected. Stay connected to your Accountability Buddies and your Support System. Stay engaged with them because your weight loss goals have to become "top of mind". There are so many things in our daily lives competing for that top position, but this journey has to be right up there. Checking in with them, seeing how they're doing, reporting your success – all of this will help you to stay motivated and inspired to keep going forward on your journey. Remember, your group is depending on you to stay committed to this process, for them, for yourself and for the reason you started in the first place.

Keep Going in Those Times When You Want to Give Up

You are going to have to hunker down like NEVER before. You are going to have to push yourself to keep going when everything in you wants to quit. You are going to have to refuse to allow yourself to give in, even when your appetite is screaming for something that is not on your plan.

I remember that I was helping out a friend in their cupcake shop when I got started. She made DELICIOUS gourmet cupcakes. Some of them would be filled with things like pudding, syrups, or other delectable items. I was setting up her shop for her daily, so I was responsible for icing the cupcakes that would be placed in the case for the day. Well, the filled cupcakes had to be cored out so that the filling could be placed in the cupcake. That meant that I had to cut the center crown of the cupcake out. Well, there was no need to waste a perfectly good piece of cake, so I spent months training my appetite to desire the core. When I started my weight loss journey, as I told you before, I was using the Shred Diet, which promised that you would lose four inches and two dress sizes in six weeks. Every time I would core out one of those cupcakes, I would say, "six weeks, four inches, two dress sizes" and toss the core in the trash. I had to continually remind myself what I was working toward. My mouth watered every time I cored those cupcakes, but I just kept telling myself what I was working towards. I knew that if I gave in, it was going to mess me up at the end of my six weeks and I wouldn't reach my four inches or my two dress sizes. I had a goal that I was working towards, and I didn't want ME to mess that up. Was it hard? YES!!! But was it worth it? ABSOLUTELY!! If I had continued eating those cored cupcake pieces, I would not be where I am today. I have come SO far, and it was because I was committed to meet my goal and to keep going in those times when I wanted to give in.

If You Mess Up...Recommit!

Have you ever been on a weight loss journey and messed up and felt like you just needed to give up? Well DON'T!!! We all mess up from time to time. We don't always get it right. It doesn't mean that we should give up all together. It just means that you messed up today, but tomorrow is a brand new day! It's filled with new opportunities to get it right, so don't give up! Keep reaching for those goals and don't stop until you reach them! Refocus, Reconnect, and Recommit!

Transparent Moment: Do you want to know the reason why I still have not reached my goal as I am writing this book? Because I got complacent. I reached my wedding size and high school dress size and I got content. I've still been losing, but yet I'm still a size 12/14. I got comfortable and wasn't really super pressed with continuing to my goal. My clothes fit nicely, I looked good again, I was out of my 16 altogether and honestly, I slacked off. Oh, I was still hitting the gym six to seven-times-a-week and sometimes two-times-a-day, but I was really only maintaining. I had started eating things that were contrary to weight loss. See, there is a saying in the fitness industry that weight loss is 80% diet, 20% exercise. I cannot lose weight without eating properly. I am happy to have been able to maintain my loss and still lose a few more pounds, but I have not reached my goal. Then, I had an injury where I tore a tendon in my ankle, so my cardio had to be cut back drastically. I could no longer do two Zumba classes a day or a Piloxing and Zumba class back to back. I was reduced to doing cycling and elliptical for cardio, and I HATED cycling when I first started. So, in a two-month period, I picked up about 10 pounds. This was very discouraging to me, and I knew I had to do something because if I continued to eat poorly and not be able to exercise, I would be well on my way to ballooning back to where I came from – and that was UNACCEPTABLE! I determined I would correct my eating habits and refocus myself so that I could go ahead and not only lose that 10 pounds, but the remaining 40 that I still had to lose. Well I did and lost another 5 in addition to that at the time of this writing.

If our mind zones out in any area – eating or exercise – then we will not reach our goals. Though weight-loss is only 20% exercise, it is necessary to achieve 100% success. Recommit. Remember why you started this journey. Think about the people you are accountable to. Reach out to your Support System for help and inspiration, and whatever you do – DON'T STOP!

Questions…

If you should happen to find yourself in a place where you feel you want to quit, or your drive has fallen off some, please revisit the reason why you started and write it here.

____

____

____

____

____

Identify what happened to cause you to fall out of focus:

How will you refocus?

Tips

Set Yourself Up for Success

You want to make sure that you set yourself up for success and not failure. What do I mean by that? I mean that if you know that chips or cookies are your weakness, then either don't have them in the house where you can easily reach for them, or choose some healthier options. There are times when we have a craving for chocolate that we just can't shake. Well, instead of reaching for high calorie milk chocolate, have dark chocolate, or instead of a candy bar, or cookie, there are lots of wholesome alternatives now you can try. You can choose granola bars that have chocolate or caramel drizzled on them from Fiber One. There are low-fat ice cream versions from companies like Weight Watchers. Even some of the major chip-manufacturing companies have low-fat or baked options. You may not like the taste of those because you've programmed your palate for the high-calorie, high-fat counterparts, but once you set your mind that these will be your new alternatives and eat them enough, you will gain a taste for them.

Think Marathon...Not Sprint

We have to change our perspective when it comes to weight loss. This weight did not come on us overnight, yet we expect that if we start working out today, we should see major results by the end of the week. Well, that's unrealistic. Doctors recommend that to lose weight safely, a person would need to lose no more than two pounds per week. So patience is the key here. Also, I've seen people that have lost a lot of weight really quickly, only to gain it back over time. I believe this is because they have not developed the necessary tools and understanding to create a disciplined mindset and retrain their appetite. Let's look at being in this for the long haul, not for a mad dash.

Take Before Pictures

You've heard my story. I was blown away by the results I saw in just three weeks. However, at the time I took the picture, I felt nothing was happening. It seemed like I wasn't losing any weight, and I was failing at this. Yet, when I took the picture, it was very obvious that there was indeed something happening! So, I always recommend that people take their picture at the beginning of their weight loss journey so that when it seems nothing is happening, you can clearly see that it is.

I also recall when I attended the ACHI Magazine Award Gala for 2014 (where I won Entrepreneur of the Year by the way), and I felt as if I was at a standstill in my weight loss. It felt as if I had reached a plateau; however, when I compared the picture that night to the one I had taken in September of 2013 (7 months into my weight loss journey), I could tell that I had truly been making progress. I was much smaller than I was in that picture.

So TAKE PICTURES of yourself, even when it feels like nothing is happening. If you are still working out, still eating correctly, still going for it, then something is happening, and pictures don't lie (at least the ones that you take with your camera anyway)!

In Times of Plateau…Change it Up!

If you find that you have truly reached a plateau and the scale is not moving, don't get discouraged. There may be times in your journey that you start losing inches more than pounds. Keep checking how your rings feel, how your clothes and coats feel. You may just be at a point where you're losing inches, especially if you've incorporated strength training in your routine.

Muscle weighs more than fat, so you may find your scale fluctuating as you add muscle. Don't get upset, muscle is a good thing. See, building muscle tone is good because when you lose weight, you lose fat, as well as muscle. So building your muscle is good as you're losing. It helps you to look leaner, since it takes up less space than fat, and it is reported to help increase your metabolism. This is good because after a weight training session, your body will go on to continue to burn calories because the speed of your metabolism has been increased. So don't be afraid to add those weights in your workout. If you have concerns about bulking up, just talk to the fitness instructor at your gym to share concerns and get advice or even a customized workout plan from them.

If you hit a plateau, change things up! Usually, that means that your body has grown accustomed to the routine that you're currently doing, so switch it up. Add strength training, do a different type of cardio, incorporate a new activity and switch things up so that you get a new set of muscles operating which will bring about some new weight loss.

Also, as it relates to women, we do retain water during our menstrual cycles; so don't be discouraged by that if you see an increase in the scale. Also be mindful if you have certain cravings during those times as well, such as chocolate or salty items. Even though the hormonal changes in your body may create increase demand for certain unhealthy items, armed with the knowledge of what is going on, you may be better able to resist those cravings.

Break Away From the Scale

I think that this may be a challenge for anyone that owns a bathroom scale that is on a weight loss journey. You do all this work, cut back on all these calories and you want to see how you're doing. It's extremely tempting to get on the scale every time you go into the bathroom. However, I would caution against this. You may have a day that the scale doesn't move, or moves up even. Again, we have all kinds of changes going on in our bodies at any given moment, so the scale could fluctuate. I suggest (as do many other health/fitness experts) that you only weigh yourself one time per week. Choose a day as your weigh-in day, and only weigh yourself that day each week. Do it at the same time of day and in the same condition. If you generally weigh yourself while in your undergarments, then do it the same way every week. Believe it or not, our clothes do add to the scale. That's why I don't get too upset when I go to the doctor and the scale is higher than my weight at home.

Dealing with Disruptions

Work projects, sickness, children's schedules, injuries; anything can come up and break our routine. It can often be hard to adjust, especially if it's for a prolonged period of time. How do you handle an unplanned disruption? The best way I have found is to have options. If you are used to going to the gym for a certain class at a certain day/time, check the gym schedule to see if the class is offered on a different day and time that will accommodate your schedule. Don't stay away too long. If you can't check in with your Accountability Buddy/group as frequently as you once did, make sure you get reconnected as soon as possible. You need that encouragement and support to keep you focused and motivated. If you have a new work schedule or have some demanding days that you have to miss your regular workout for a while, be sure to get some fitness in during another time. Can you do something at home, like a video, bike ride or one of the interactive videos (Wii or Xbox)? Take a walk on your lunch break.

Switch things up and try a new class. Pick up a new video from the store that you can do at home. Whatever you do, you cannot allow the disruptions to disrupt you. You have to be committed to this journey, not just to a class or a workout. Be flexible and see this as an opportunity to try something new.

When I had my injury with the torn tendon, I knew I had to keep going or else it would be detrimental. I absolutely adore my group exercise classes like Zumba and Piloxing, but while I was healing, I had to do something that would not have all the pounding that those classes had. So, I had to go back and remember some of the things I did before those classes became so dominant in my workout routine. I did the elliptical machine that I can burn a lot of calories on. I started riding the recumbent bike just to give me some variety. I usually did both of these machines on the manual setting, however one morning I switched up the bike routine and added a program that included random hills. I had it set at level 15. I was NOT ready for what I was about to experience! I was huffing and puffing trying to get up those hills. My heart was pumping like it was going to come right out of my chest. I lowered the levels down until I eventually got to around level nine. When I got off that bike, I felt amazing! All the muscles in my lower extremities had been worked. They were engaged and alert! It was amazing! I was won after that. I also incorporated my strength training three days a week. Even though I wasn't able to get the calorie burn that I usually was able to get through my cardio group classes, I still wanted to make sure I was staying active while I recuperated. I also began to add Pilates in as well, as this is a great exercise to help lengthen and tone your muscles and give you that lean dancer body. Many of these alternative workouts I had forgotten about, so even though the injury was a bad thing, it was working for my good. I saw results from the changes that I began to make within the first couple of weeks.

Disruptions are a part of life. Things don't always go according to plan. However you have to have a contingency plan in place as well. You have to be willing to do some things that you may not have done before or not even liked before to keep making progress in this journey. In the face of disruptions, stay active and keep moving, making the necessary adjustments to ensure your continued success.

Make it a Family Affair

In February 2013, we did not have a gym membership. So when it was time to begin getting active, we started walking around our neighborhood. We live in a large community with several different developments. We would walk through them, varying our course to keep some variety in our routine. To challenge ourselves, we would walk a little farther each time. We would take our daughter with us, and she would ride her bike sometimes while we walked. She and I would ride our bikes together. We would play the interactive games on our Wii. We had dance games and exercise videos, and we would motivate each other that way. These are the exercises we did while we were on the Shred Diet. During that time, I lost 18 pounds and my husband lost 21. This was fun for our family and we got to bond and spend quality time together. About three months into our weight loss journey, my husband renewed our membership to the YMCA, and that's when I started the group exercise classes. So, even if you don't have money for a gym membership or time to go to a gym, or don't like the gym setting, there are still plenty of things that you can do at home with your family to get exercise. There are days when I will still go for a walk, pop in a workout video, or do a video game to change up my routine, or if I couldn't make it to a class.

Addressing Objections

Often times when I do a seminar or speak at a conference about starting an eating regimen or working out, I will get some objections as to why people don't start. I want to address a few of the more popular concerns here:

I don't want to mess up my hair

I am natural, meaning my hair is not chemically processed, so I don't worry about destroying a $60 hairstyle. However, there are many ladies that do. So, I reached out to a stylist that I know, Yolanda Woods, of Hair PhD in Portsmouth, Virginia. I reached out to her because she works out avidly as well. She stated that she often tells people to keep their hair wrapped while they are working out, and if they workout in the evening, they need to allow the hair to dry before combing it down. She also stated that Sew-in hair weaves have become very popular with clients that want to work out. She stated that braids and up dos are also great alternatives. She cautioned that clients should try to shampoo their hair every week as the salt from the sweat can be drying to the hair.

I don't have time to workout

The problem is that often times we view exercise as an option. We can choose whether or not we will work out. We have to change our perspective to view it as a priority. We have to constantly have it on our minds. We have to plan our workout times. It must become a necessary part of our day, just like brushing our teeth or going to work. It must become a part of our lives. So, when you go to the store, you park a little farther to get a little more walking in for the day (10,000 steps is the minimum required). If we go in a store that has two entrances, choose the side that is opposite of the items you need. Get up 30 minutes earlier so you can get in some exercise. Take 30 minutes of your lunch break to go for a walk and the other 30 to eat. Go for a bike ride or walk after dinner. Do some squats or sit-ups while you're cooking dinner or watching a television show. Do some chair dips on this side of your bed or tub while you're waiting for your water to heat up for your shower. You'd be surprised at how much time we actually waste in a day. One hour is 4% of your day. You can find that time, even if you break it up into small increments. With running a ministry with four different brands, planning events, servicing clients, managing a household, spending time with my daughter, producing a talk show, and helping out affiliate ministries, I am extremely busy, but I understand that my health and my goals are a priority, so ensuring that I make time to work out every day is important. My health and fitness are on the top of my mind for me, and to be successful, it must be for you, too.

I don't have time to plan my foods

As stated in the previous example, you would be surprised at the time you actually have in a day or a week. You can plan your meals while you're driving. If you have a smart phone, or a recording device, you can plan while you're driving to work. When you're cooking dinner, you can plan your meals. If you walk for 30 minutes during lunch, then you can eat your lunch during the other 30 and plan your meals while you're eating. Where there is a will, there is a way! We find all the time in the world to do the things we enjoy doing, so we can find time to do the things we need to do as well.

Eating healthy is too expensive

I understand this one well because it is taxing on the bank account; healthy foods do seem to cost a little more than readily accessible junk food. However, a part of this new lifestyle is developing discipline. One thing that you can do is use coupons. If there are household products vying for a major spot in the budget, then use coupons for those things. You could even take a class and learn how to become an "extreme couponer". People are buying products that cost hundreds of dollars, but only paying pennies for them. That would then free up your budget to purchase healthy foods for your family as well as other things you need for your life. Learning to save money is never a bad thing! Think about it this way: in the long run, a poor diet will end up costing you more money in prescriptions, insurance, doctor bills, etc. Pay now and have a great quality of life or pay later *and* have a poor quality of life; either way, we pay. I feel we may as well enjoy life in the process.

I don't know how to prepare healthy meals

So if you didn't grow up in an environment where healthy cooking was done, then you may only know how to prepare dishes according to the way you grew up. Well, that's no longer an excuse. There are tons and tons and tons of healthy recipes that are available online and in cookbooks. You can do that during the time that you're surfing the Internet at work. (Oops, did I just say that?)

******

At the end of the day, if we will be honest with ourselves, all of these objections are just excuses—legitimate concerns—but still excuses. If we really want to do something and it's really a priority, we will make the necessary adjustments to figure out how to go around the objections to achieve our goals. So the last key I will give you is this: ELIMINATE THE EXCUSES! If it is a priority, you will figure out how to get it done. Now, the challenge is to make it a priority in your life.

Tools/Equipment

Here are some tools/equipment that you may need to help you as you embark upon your weight loss journey:

Pedometer

A pedometer tracks your steps per day, and your goal should be around 10,000 steps per day. That seems like a lot, but you don't realize how many steps are required to go to various destinations; whether it is in your house, to the mailbox, in your office, etc. When you're wearing a pedometer, it makes you more conscious to take more steps throughout your day. It will encourage you to park farther away from the grocery store, or to take the steps instead of the elevator, to take the dog for more or longer walks, or get up and move from your desk. Adding those extra steps in your day help you to get meet your steps goal for each day, and helps you get healthier in the process.

You can purchase a pedometer from retail stores like Wal-Mart or Walgreens, or you can go online and purchase from amazon.com or ebay.com.

Calorie Counter

Specifically, these are devices worn on your arm or wrist that track the amount of calories you burn through the day, or during a specific exercise. These are great because they more accurately show the calories you burn than an app on your phone or your gym may do. These only give an approximation on what you've burned, but the calorie tracker gives a more accurate report. Knowing what you've burned will help you determine which exercise you need to do to meet your specific goal, which exercises are most effective, and help you feel a great sense of accomplishment seeing how much your hard work and effort is paying off.

Again, retailers such as Wal-Mart will have these, and online at amazon.com and ebay.com are great options as well.

MP3 Player or Phone & Headphones

If you do not have a smartphone, you will at least need an mp3 player and headphones for your workouts. If you start off walking in your neighborhood or you decide to go right into the gym and get on the treadmill or hit the weights, having music that motivates and appeals to you will be an asset in your journey. You may even want to have motivational sayings, movies, or whatever you prefer to help you pass the time while you are exercising. You will need these items to do that. Some gyms also have machines with televisions on them. I need my headphones on these machines because I am not really a machine person. I enjoy group exercise classes like Zumba, cycling, etc. The machines don't engage me like those classes, so I need something to help take my mind off the fact that I am exercising. (Did I just say that out loud?) Even though most gyms and fitness centers will offer "community" headphones, I prefer my own for sanitary reasons.

Again, you can visit the retailers mentioned earlier, as well as those such as Target or Best Buy.

Armband to Hold mp3 Player

You may also invest in an armband to hold your phone or mp3 player. This will free your hands while you are working out.

You can purchase these fairly inexpensively at amazon.com, but you can visit other retailers mentioned here as well.

Workout Attire

My husband always says you workout better when you feel like you look good. Many times we think "workout" and we just throw on anything. However, I would encourage you to invest in some good, quality workout gear. It will help motivate you, and it builds your confidence and self-esteem. When we are just starting to work out, we may be in a place of not feeling that great about ourselves, but if we look good while working out, it may help to boost that confidence. Not only that, but it helps us to gauge our progress. We can tell where we were when we started and three months down the line; we should see some improvement in how these clothes fit. (Ideally, they should be getting a little looser.)

There are tons of retailers out there where you can purchase attire. Also, you're always welcome to get some inspirational Fitness Finesse w/ Rae wear from our Fitness Finesse Shop at our website. Visit www.miraenter prises.info and click on Fitness Finesse to view our selections.

Proper Tennis Shoes for Your Exercise

I cannot stress the importance of this enough! You have to know your feet. Do you walk normal; do you supinate, or over pronate? What exercise will you be doing? Using one pair of tennis shoes for all activities will not work. There are shoes you will need for running, another pair for cross training, a different pair for Zumba, etc. You also have to know what shoes will give your feet the best support. How do I know all this? I've had to learn it the hard way! Knee pain from wearing the wrong shoes in Zumba, torn shoes from not having the insole support due to the fact that I supinate (my feet roll out), plantar fasciitis from the wrong shoes and lack of support and the "Big Papa" of them all, a torn Peroneal tendon in my left ankle, from a lack of proper foot support. Trust me, you need the right shoes! Do your research, find out if you supinate, over pronate, or walk normal. Talk to your podiatrist; get help from informed tennis shoe retailers. Do what you must to ensure that your feet will be protected as much as possible as you workout. Your feet are your foundation, and they take a tremendous amount of pounding when we exercise. Do what you need to in order to ensure that they will continue to function properly and be comfortable to avoid injury in your body. An injury is counterproductive to a workout regimen, and could throw you way off in your efforts, so be sure to give your feet the love they need so they can continue to produce for you!

Videos and/or Video Games

If you plan on working out at home, these are great, and can be purchased at any of the retailers mentioned above

Food Intake Tracker

Keeping track of your food intake is crucial to your success as well. Some people use a journal to record what they have eaten throughout the day. Personally, I prefer to plan my meals which helps give me more discipline in my meal choices. I've created a Nutrition & Exercise Planner that I use to plan my meals each day. I explain it in detail in the next section.

How to Use the 30 Day Exercise & Nutrition Planner

There is an adage that I fully subscribe to that says, "If you fail to plan, you plan to fail". I have found that when I fail to plan, I fail!

I have created the planner/journal and it is available for purchase at Amazon.com. This planner will be beneficial in helping you plan out your meals and exercise ahead of time. I find it serves as a road map for me. I don't see these meals as suggestions; I view them as my directives. This is how I have to operate, and if I don't, I find myself at mealtime saying, "What do I feel like?" or "What do I have a taste for?" Those are the times I get into trouble. I have to discipline myself to plan my meal and stick to the plan.

I found that planning works best when I do it for the week, so I set time aside on Sunday morning or evening to do it. If you cannot do it then, doing it daily is an option as well. Just make sure you take time to do it. You will be surprised at how empowering it is to plan your exercise and nutrition ahead of time!

Meals/Snacks

On the planner, you will find four options for Meals. Many diet and nutrition experts recommend that we should eat several small meals per day, every three to four hours to keep your metabolism revved up. So, this is what the planner is based on. It also provides a slot for the time that you will eat the meal. I have found this to be very helpful in keeping me disciplined and on track. There are also slots available for you to plan your snacks. I don't know about you, but this is crucial for me! Snacking is a problem for me. I tend to get a little carried away with the snacking if I don't use my planner. I plan my snacks ahead of time so that I know what I will be having that day to keep me on task.

Water Intake

There are eight spaces for water intake. Between six to eight glasses of water daily has been the amount of water that we have heard for years that we needed to drink. However, I recently read an article written by holistic nutritionist, Yuri Elkaim in which he stated that in order to avoid dehydration; we need to drink half our body weight in ounces just to simply function. He goes on to state that if we are active (working out, hiking, etc.), that we need to add another liter, or four cups to that amount.[2]

So, let's give an example:

If a person weighs 200 pounds currently, then his/her normal water intake that his/her body needs in order to function properly would be 100 ounces, which is equivalent to 12.5 cups of water. If he/she began exercising and sweating profusely, then he/she would need to add one liter, or four cups of water to that amount. Therefore, he/she would need to drink 15.6 cups of water per day.

So, as it relates to our water spaces on our Planner, the person in our example should double up on the cups of water he/she drinks during each water drinking session. So,

---

[2] Elkaim, Y. (2013, September 13). The truth about how much water you should really drink: your hydration questions, answered. *U.S. News & World Report.* Retrieved from http://health.usnews.com/health-news/blogs/eat-run/2013/09/13/the-truth-about-how-much-water-you-should-really-drink

for Glass #1 at 5am, drink two glasses as opposed to simply drinking one. That will ensure that he/she is getting the appropriate amount of water his/her body needs.

Water intake is extremely important to our overall health and it hydrates our organs and cells, cushions our joints, and removes waste through our bodies, so we need to ensure that we are getting adequate amounts of water daily. Use this chart to ensure that you are drinking at the appropriate times and amounts.

Steps

There is a space here for your steps. The goal every day should be around 10K steps. You can use this space to record what your steps were for the day so that you can be mindful of the need to increase your steps throughout your day.

Get Up & Move (G.U.A.M.)

We need to move throughout the day. Even if we exercise, research has shown that sitting down at a desk all day may be hazardous to our health. A report on *The Today* show stated that "sitting too much is the new smoking"[3], going on to state that it raises the risk of diabetes, heart disease, and cancer. Not only that, but the risk increases with every two-hour-period of sitting time. In addition, having a workout routine before or after work does not help in alleviating the risks.

So we need to GET UP & MOVE (GUAM)! The spaces

---

[3] Holohan, M. (2014, June 16). Don't let sitting all day kill you – 5 easy ways to keep moving at your desk. *Today Health.* Retrieved from (http://www.today.com/health/dont-let-sitting-all-day-kill-you-5-easy-ways-1D79812002

are here to record the times when you will get up from your desk and move. You have to plan these times or else they will not happen! There are seven slots here, so that's one time-per-hour you should be getting up, walking around the office, doing some squats, doing desk push-ups, walking the stairs, standing up or doing something that will increase your heart rate and get the blood pumping. The next time you need to send an email to a co-worker, why not walk to their desk and tell them instead?

Set 10 minutes out of each hour to G.U.A.M. So maybe at :50 of every hour, that's your time to move, or maybe at 10 minutes after, that's your time. If you establish a set unit of time to do it, that will make it become more of a habit for you.

Today's Workout

This section is for you to plan your workout for the day. Determine in the morning what your workout will be for the day, or plan your workouts for the week on Sunday. This is a good time to plan to try a new workout that you've been considering. Put it down on your planner, and you will stand a better chance of actually doing it. Planning your workout in advance helps you to get into the mindset that you're not going to do what you feel like doing, you're doing what you've planned to do.

I keep my sheet for the day open so that I have it before me and I can check my times of everything I need to be doing, i.e. water, meal, G.U.A.M., etc. That way I can take a quick peek and know where I need to be.

30 Day Exercise & Nutrition Planner & Journal

Meals

Meal #1:

Time: ________

Meal: ______________________________________

Snack #1: ____________________

Meal #2:

Time: ________

Meal: ______________________________________

Snack #2: ____________________

Meal #3:

Time: ________

Meal: ______________________________________

Snack #3: ____________________

Meal #4:

Time: ________

Meal: ______________________________________

Water:

Glass #1:
Glass #2:
Glass #3:
Glass #4:
Glass #5:
Glass #6:
Glass #7:
Glass #8:

Steps:

____

Get Up & Move:
Time #1: _______
Time #2: _______
Time #3: _______
Time #4: _______
Time #5: _______
Time #6: _______
Time #7: _______

Today's Workout:

Cardio: _______________
Cardio: _______________
Strength: _____________

Goals today:

Motivation:

Feelings/Challenges:

Accomplishments/Improvements Needed:

Conclusion

My goal with this book is to help you gain insight into some of the necessary elements that help support your weight-loss goals. I personally have always known that I needed to eat "right" and exercise, but this has been a journey of discovery for me. I have come to realize some really important keys to achieving weight-loss success that I never knew before. I personally am so grateful to have learned them, and I am extremely grateful to all the people that have played an important role in this process with me.

You CAN do this! If you implement the keys introduced in this book, you will find yourself winning in your weight-loss journey. This is possible, and I have every confidence in you! If you do these things, there will be nothing stopping you from making this time the time you reach your weight-loss goals!

Please contact me via our website, www.miraenterprises.info, and let me know how your journey is going. I also invite you to join the Fitness Finesse w/Rae Accountability Group on Facebook. We are a group of individuals that are on the journey to reaching our goals and celebrating our successes together. You don't have to go it alone, you can connect with a group of likeminded individuals that are on the same journey as you are, that will support, inspire, motivate, encourage and cheer you on to your victory.

You CAN do this!!!

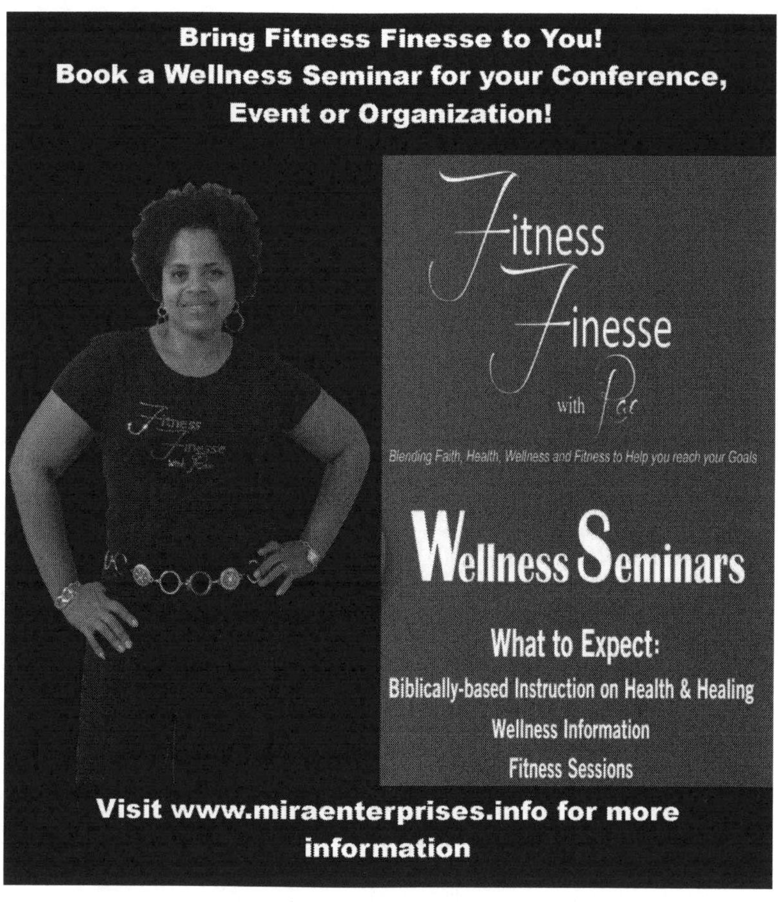

Bring Fitness Finesse to You!
Book a Wellness Seminar for your Conference, Event or Organization!
Fitness Finesse
with
Blending Faith, Health, Wellness and Fitness to Help you reach your Goals
Wellness Seminars
What to Expect:
Biblically-based Instruction on Health & Healing
Wellness Information
Fitness Sessions
Visit www.miraenterprises.info for more information

Made in the USA
Middletown, DE
23 April 2015